A Healthy Way to Lose Weight

By Ben Granger

Use these Steps and you will have weight loss guaranteed.

Perspective

1. Your mind has a perspective, and your body has a perspective.

2. To change your body's perspective, do not restrict, train it, by giving your body the foods it needs, and teaching at the same time to burn fat.

3. All foods are made of nutrients; it is your proportions, and your overall lifestyle, that influences how your body uses them.

Training

1. Your body will change into a system that is healthy if you contribute healthy foods and nutrients, and limit calories by giving it less food and not a complete restriction.

2. You need protein, and other vitamins to maintain a healthy body which contributes to a healthy weight, that is why starvation is not truly effective.

Weight Loss

1. If you use BPM, you will see results, because it is a system that develops what your body needs to stay healthy and active, and losing weight without much restriction of anything in your diet.

2. Weight loss is a gradual and natural and is simply a reflection that you are maintaining your system in way that it will lose weight. It is a reflection of a healthy perspective and a healthier diet.

The Secret Steps

1. Do not eat a big or grand size lunch, I cannot stress this enough, do not eat a large high calorie lunch, and drink water or low calorie tea or milk, and not a soft drink such as coke.

2. Completely cut out sugary drinks such as Coca Cola or others like it, the sugar content is quickly converted to fat, not only stopping you from losing real weight, but also lowering your energy level, clogging and overworking your intestines, and even making you prone to hypertension and diabetes in the long run.

3. Food is not your enemy, it is not about how much food you eat, but how you train your system to handle the fat, of course eating more food in the long run, reprogram's your metabolic rate and your ability to burn fat by changing your metabolism. The secret is to skip a meal particularly lunch, so your system will be updated to burn the fat more often. If you do not send the message to burn fat more often by not being active, and eating more without creating a limitation, your body will never be trained well enough to burn the fat, and gain calories that it need for energy.

4. Eating food is ok; it is not about starvation, or totally restraining yourself, from food. It is about simple everyday lifestyle changes, that can you help you in the long run gain more energy, and develop better health, which overall contributes to weight loss.

5. Gaining weight is not a discouragement, it is simply a reflection of changes you are making in your lifestyle, and the nutrients you are putting into your body.

Fat is not an evil blob that many would like to believe, it is actually a very important component in my aspects of your body, in fact your body would never sustain itself without fat cells.

6. Changes you make in your lifestyle, influence how your nutrients work together in your body, which overall contributes to fat loss in the body. It is lifestyle, lifestyle, lifestyle, not restriction.

7. Do not cut out the important that patterns of your life to lose weight, especially sleep. Sleep is a very important to the body's overall energy and functioning, and also to the immune system, do not cut sleep out of your diet in a attempt to weight, just train your body to burn more fat by skipping a meal a day, eat only half your meals, and have water and diet drinks.

8. Drink more water, if you drink water that cleanses your body, and fuels nutrients, causing you to lose much more weight if you combine it with the constant reprogramming that you are skipping a meal.

9. Do not do it to gain a great six pack, or to impress people. Great abs can take months and even years of strength training and although are a reflection of a healthy body, they are not a goal everyone should set, just to lose weight. Workout and run or swim to lose gradually over time. Self-confidence is gained by making small changes, which can lead to big change overtime.

10. Gain a fresh healthy perspective, do not consistently think about losing weight all the time, just make small changes, and do not ever get obsessed, and you could see results that I did.

Remember

- The formula is to train by changing your lifestyle habits, not creating a total restriction of food that never works.

- Even though restricting food can cause you to lose weight, it the cycle that your body needs to stay in a healthy condition, which can hurt you in the long run, and many times causes people to end up in the hospital.

- Do not fall for fad diets, use your common sense, and train your body to be healthy by making small positive changes. If those diets actually worked for everyone, then we all have six pack abs, and a great body. Do not fall for any fad diets, no matter how chemically effective they might sound.

- Drink healthy drinks, and not sodas. Having a soda is once a while is completely ok, but use your common sense, and do not drink them consistently throughout the day. Sodas are chemically structured by caffeine to give an artificial energy, that keeps you awake, but it does not make you any healthier so that you lose weight, and sugar is a contributor to diabetes and heart disease, so drink healthy drinks.

- If you really want to get a well-defined body or great abs, losing weight is only about half the component to it, you need strength training, and also a constant diet of healthy protein. Many people never develop a six pack, even following a completely healthy regimen. So you should it make your goal to lose weight, to gain.

a healthier body in the long run, not just for the great six pack.

- You can still eat some of the food you enjoy. It about making a positive healthy new prospective on your diet, not a complete restriction of foods you like to eat.

- Remember if you train your body to be healthier, then it will get healthier over time, causing a natural weight loss. A complete restriction does not train your body, it only breaks the cycle, which can still lead to weight loss, but not necessary to a healthy body.

- Weight and fat is not evil, it is a great overall reflection of your body is changing, and how it is handling nutrients and fat, by your energy levels, and your overall lifestyle. Change your perspective and make your body more alert and productive by burning calories and fat, by simply limiting a meal, such as lunch, and then eating half of your meals the rest of the day.

- Nobody's perfect, if your body still is not losing weight, even after restricting some calories from your diet, then just attempt to keep a healthy perspective.

- Last tip; use the body perspective method that I have used to lose weight.

Body Perspective Method

1. Give you body an edge of time to know that it can burn more fat by skipping 13 lunch and only eating half your meals after that time.

2. Program your body to make more protein and less fat, by eating a protein meal, but only eating half of it, instead of the whole meal, that way your body, will train to consume and store protein, and burn more fat.

3. Your proportions of food, train your system to handle nutrients and fat, if you eat a diet high in protein, and only a small meal, then your body will know to take in more protein, and you will lose weight.

4. Eat foods that make your body healthy, but do not completely restrict foods you like, because it is about small gradual changes. That is about all I have for this book, but another helpful guide many come out in the future after this one.

Plans to Reach a Healthy Weight

Introduction to the Plan

My plan for losing weight is simple and effective, and helps you shed pounds, quick and easily, without over straining yourself, it is a simple daily process that you follow each and every day of the week. First here is how the plan works, you must eat foods high in protein, low in bad crabs, and moderate in good crabs. Second, you must do some simple exercises the will not exhaust you, this includes setups, crunches, and leg ups. Also you can perform these exercises on the couch as well. I followed this plan, and I actually when from 175 pounds to 135 pounds in 8 months, it is incredible. The plan is extremely simple, just cut out foods high in bad crabs, and completely cut out sugar, I mean do not drink regular sodas, and switch to diet drinks instead, and do setups and crunches, at least 3 to 5 times a week, believe me you will see a dramatic improvement, in your weight, and your health.

The Eating Plan

Follow this plan at Least 5 days a week

- Breakfast- Eat breakfast foods, that are low in bad crabs, moderate in good crabs, and high in protein, this includes sausage, eggs, cereal, grits, oatmeal, wheat bread, and you can even at bacon. You can drink orange juice, and other kinds of fruit drinks, that low in bad crabs, and no-natural sugar. Do not consume soft drinks that are high in high-fructose syrup, or bad crabs during or after breakfast. You can drink a diet soda for breakfast, if you want to. Foods you should not eat for breakfast; include pancakes, waffles, French toast, pizza, or pigs in a blanket.

- Lunch- Lunch should consumed in moderation, foods that you should, eat for lunch, include those are low in bad crabs, and high in protein. This includes, a ham or turkey sandwich, you can add what you like to it, but I recommend you cut mayonnaise, a salad, chicken, a chicken sandwich on a wheat bun. Foods you should not eat for lunch, includes hot dogs, corn dogs, and milkshakes.

- Dinner- For dinner, you can eat meal that is high in protein, and high in good crabs, but low in bad crabs. This includes steak, shrimp, chicken, and pork. Foods you should not eat for dinner, include anything fast food, nothing from McDonalds, Hardees, etc. The Exercise Plan.

- Morning- You does not have to do an over-strenuous workout in the morning, I recommend you do at least. Do 50 to 80 setups if you can and also run for at least 30.

minutes, this will leaving feeling healthier, and may help shed one or two pounds.

- Afternoon- Do 50 to 100 setups, if you can, it is not necessary to run in the afternoon, but you can if you please. Do at least 20 to 50 crunches, and try leg ups as well.

- Evening- Exercise is not necessary in the evening, if you already completed the steps in the morning, and afternoon.

- Night- Get a good rest, period.

Six Pack Abs Guide

Gaining six pack abs, takes patience and time to achieve, but following this helpful guide, may help you in achieving a great set of abs. Getting six pack abs is two step processes, first you must strengthen your abdominal muscles, and lose body fat. Although losing body fat may seem like a simple process, it does time much dedication and effort, willpower, patience and time, but once you achieve it, it is definitely worth it.

The Steps

1. The first step in getting a six pack, is you must change your diet, a golden rule to building a great set of abs, is no matter, how many setups and crunches that you do, you must maintain a healthy diet, which includes eating fruits, vegetables, meats, and chicken. You can do setups and crunches, until you turn blue, but if you do not change your diet, you will not see any change in your physique. The diet that you must follow in order to gain a six pack is low on bad crabs, moderate on good crabs, and you must, if you can, completely cut out processed sugar. Combining a healthy diet, with regular exercise, will help you get on your way, to a better-looking body.

2. The second major step, in gaining a six pack, is doing exercises, although just changing your diet alone, will you help become healthier, and is a major factor in developing a six pack, you must exercise regularly. Cardio, setups, and crunches, are all exercises, that help to create well- defined abs. Setups, will help to burn off the excess body fat, that must be lost, in order to see your abs. Cardio exercises, including running, jogging, and just walking, will help to burn the reserve fat, that covers your abs. Crunches, will help to tighten your abs, and make them further come out. Also lifting weights will develop and strengthen your abs, as well.

3. The third step in getting a six pack, is you must be cautious about what you are eating throughout the day, overloading, on bad crabs, fats, and sugar, will absolutely ruin a six pack. These things chemically change the programming in your body by screwing.

with your hormones, and will actually cause your stomach to stop tightening. In your order for you to get a six pack, your stomach must stay tightened, and this unfortunately this cannot be maintained, if you overload on any those three things, anytime during the day.

4. Another important step, is to focus on being healthy, and maintaining a healthy weight, and have patience, and perseverance. Having a six pack, is about staying healthy and in shape, do not put all of your attention, on having the most ripped tightened abs, a great set of six pack abs, comes with total patience, and time, and does take a lot of dedication to attain.

10 Tips to Losing Weight Perspective

1. Your mind has a perspective, and your body has a perspective.

2. To change your body's perspective, do not restrict, train it, by giving your body the foods it needs, and teaching at the same time to burn fat.

3. All foods are made of nutrients; it is your proportions, and your overall lifestyle, that influences how your body uses them.

Training

1. Your body will change into a system that is healthy if you contribute healthy foods and nutrients, and limit calories by giving it less food, and not a complete restriction.

2. You need protein, and other vitamins to maintain a healthy body which contributes to a healthy weight, that is why starvation is not truly effective.

Weight Loss

1. If you use BPM, you will see results, because it is a system that develops what your body needs to stay healthy and active, and losing weight without much restriction of anything in your diet. Weight loss is a gradual and natural and is simply a reflection that you are maintaining your system in way that it will lose weight. It is reflection of a healthy perspective and a healthier diet.

The Secret Steps

1. Do not eat a big or grand size lunch, I cannot stress this enough, do not eat a large high calorie lunch, and drink water or low calorie tea or milk, and not a soft drink such as coke.

2. Completely cut out sugary drinks such as Coca Cola or others like it, the sugar content is quickly converted to fat, not only stopping you from losing real weight, but also lowering your energy level, clogging and overworking your intestines, and even making you prone to hypertension and diabetes in the long run.

3. Food is not your enemy, it is not about how much food you eat, but how you train your system to handle the fat, of course eating more food in the long run, reprogram's your metabolic rate and your ability to burn fat by changing your metabolism. The secret is to skip a meal particularly lunch, so your system will be updated to burn the fat more often. If you do not send the message to burn fat more often by not being active, and eating more without creating a limitation, your body will never be trained well enough to burn the fat, and gain calories that it need for energy.

4. Eating food is ok; it is not about starvation, or totally restraining yourself, from food. It is about simple everyday lifestyle changes, that can you help you in the long run gain more energy, and develop better health, which overall contributes to weight loss.

5. Gaining weight is not a discouragement, it is simply a reflection of changes you are making in your lifestyle, and the nutrients you are putting into your body.

how they are being put to use. Fat is not an evil blob that many would like to believe, it is actually a very important component in my aspects of your body, in fact your body would never sustain itself without fat cells. That changes your make in your lifestyle, influence how your nutrients work together in your body, which overall contributes to fat loss in the body. It is lifestyle, lifestyle, lifestyle, not restriction.

6. Do not cut out the important that patterns of your life to lose weight, especially sleep. Sleep is a very important to the body's overall energy and functioning, and also to the immune system, do not cut sleep out of your diet in a attempt to weight, just train your body to burn more fat by skipping a meal a day, eat only half your meals, and have water and diet drinks.

7. Drink more water, if you drink water that cleanses your body, and fuels nutrients, causing you to lose much more weight if you combine it with the constant reprogramming that you are skipping a meal.

8. Do not do it to gain a great six pack, or to impress people. Great abs can take months and even years of strength training and although are a reflection of a healthy body, they are not a goal everyone should set, just to lose weight. Workout and run or swim to lose gradually over time. Self-confidence is gained by making small changes, which can lead to big change overtime.

9. Gain a fresh healthy perspective, do not consistently think about losing weight all the time, just make small changes, and do not ever get obsessed, and you could see results that I did.

Remember

- The Formula is to train by changing your lifestyle habits, not creating a total restriction of food that never works.

- Even though restricting food can cause you to lose weight, it the cycle that your body needs to stay in a healthy condition, which can hurt you in the long run, and many times causes people to end up in the hospital.

- Do not fall for fad diets, use your common sense, and train your body to be healthy by making small positive changes. If those diets actually worked for everyone, then we all have six pack abs, and a great body. Do not fall for any fad diets, no matter how chemically effective they might sound.

- Drink healthy drinks, and not sodas. Having a soda is once a while is completely ok, but use your common sense, and do not drink them consistently throughout the day. Sodas are chemically structured by caffeine to give an artificial energy, that keeps you awake, but it does not make you any healthier so that you lose weight, and sugar is a contributor to diabetes and heart disease, so drink healthy drinks.

- If you really want to get a well-defined body or great abs, losing weight is only about half the component to it, you need strength training, and also a constant diet of healthy protein. Many people never develop a six pack, even following a completely healthy regimen. So you should it make your goal to lose weight, to gain.

a healthier body in the long run, not just for the great six pack.

- You can still eat some of the food you enjoy. It about making a positive healthy new prospective on your diet, not a complete restriction of foods you like to eat. Remember if you train your body to be healthier, then it will get healthier over time, causing a natural weight loss. A complete restriction does not train your body, it only breaks the cycle, which can still lead to weight loss, but not necessary to a healthy body.

- Weight and fat is not evil, it is a great overall reflection of your body is changing, and how it is handling nutrients and fat, by your energy levels, and your overall lifestyle. Change your perspective and make your body more alert and productive by burning calories and fat, by simply limiting a meal, such as lunch, and then eating half of your meals the rest of the day.

- Nobody's perfect, if your body still is not losing weight, even after restricting some calories from your diet, then just attempt to keep a healthy perspective.

- Last tip; use the body perspective method that I have used to lose weight.

Body Perspective Method

1. Give you body an edge of time to know that it can burn more fat, by skipping lunch, and only eating half your meals after that time.

2. Program your body to make more protein and less fat, by eating a protein meal, but only eating half of it, instead of the whole meal, that way your body, will train to consume and store protein, and burn more fat.

3. Your proportions of food, train your system to handle nutrients and fat, if you eat a diet high in protein, and only a small meal, then your body will know to take in more protein, and you will lose weight.

4. Eat foods that make your body healthy, but do not completely restrict foods you like, because it is about small gradual changes. Use these Steps and you will have weight loss guaranteed.

About Me

Benjamin Granger- Author

This is my short bio about myself, Benjamin Granger. Most people call me Ben, but Benjamin is my real name and my full name is Benjamin Park Granger.

I was born in Pensacola, FL on March, 28th, 1987. I also have two older siblings, one is a teacher and a city planner, and my other brother is a doctor of Physical Therapy. I was born with the skill to write quite well, and I am also a good speaker as well. Although I have not been signed to a major publisher yet, I am praying and hoping this could be my chance. I am also a researcher of historic and prehistoric documents, and I recently earned a college degree.

Throughout most of my life, I had aspirations about being good at something, and I believe that dream might be a reality. I cannot say am the greatest writer in the world, but I would love it if my books did get great recognition for my skill and talent.

My previous writing credits include a weight loss book, a history paperback book, and a book on better studying habits, an ancestral lineage book, and one other historical manuscript. I also worked on a very short story once that I did complete half-way, and I also have experience doing essays, and a few stories as a child, and am also considering a writing career in journalism.

My influences come from simply being fascinated with nature and the world around us, which is what, inspired two of my books, and I also have a lot of sci-fi, action, and some horror, which was inspiration behind my second book. I also love writing, because it helps to release the creative energy in my mind, and it is hard to stop. Am also very fascinated with the unknown and how it mixes and contours with natural and everyday circumstances, and how we can be both amazed by it, but also entertained and moved but its energy and dramatic flow.

Most of my influences come from movies and some from real life, but I include a mixture of the two in my stories. I am not setting out to be a perfect writer, but am setting out to make books, that people will enjoy for a lifetime, and I hope that you will enjoy them too.

I wrote Network Twilight, from a few different mysteries that I took a glimpse of as a kid, like Murder She Wrote, and also some sci-fi shows, like The Outer Limits. The other two books are purely based on my creative thoughts, but they included common themes, such as Star Trek, and also Battle star Galactic type stuff in 2020 Mars, and in I, Bear, I take a classic symbol and turn it into both rude and spiritual awakening for a rural community. Please review my work, and you will enjoy it. Thanks.

In conclusion, am a native Pensacola, born to two wonderful parents, and my father was a navy storekeeper, and my mother was once an accountant. I have two brothers, who have greatly succeeded in their careers, and I hope that I will be a success as well, not just in writing, but hopefully many aspirations throughout my life.

I really hope that you have enjoyed the book, a Healthy Way to Lose Weight. The book is based on my plan for weight loss, and please takes time to exercise, and eat right, before starting any diet plan, including mine, and relax, and enjoy life while doing it.